MILLION DOLLAR MORNING

Design your morning in a wholesome way

By:- Raj Aryan Purohit

INTRODUCTION

Its been years I read a quote on a book titled **"The Leader who have no Title"** by Robin Sharma, it said, **"People are awarded in public what they practice many years in private".** From that, I learned one thing that one needs to develop some set of daily rituals that he can follow every day which will lead him to a path of immense success.

So, with this book I came before you with a wonderful idea about how you can rule your day, the trick is simple you just need to rule your morning!

How can we rule our morning when we face problems to even defeat our alarm like I said before we need to follow some rule that I'm going to suggest which will help you win your morning and also your day.

Before I start the first chapter I would like to share a short experience which led me to the idea of this book.

Winters are lazy for all, who wants to leave their mattress and go out to the hard world and start their day, well I was among those lazy sloth, its not that I did overnight work and its difficult for me to wake up in morning, no I'm a student and like always I used to complete my studies till 11-11:30, then bed. Mornings were too hard to wake up, for which the rest of the day went lethargic. I hated that I wanted to change this, I went online saw videos and read many books, it interested me, I started noting down things. I felt why not to collect all these shattered pieces and make out the puzzle, I knew it will help many people like me out there. I collected information for six months also implemented them on myself and I can say, now I wake up every morning 5 am and does my rituals (*Those morning rituals that I am going to share with you in the coming chapters*). Now I'm happier than before, healthier than before and sharper than before.

It helped me and I hope it will help rest of the world too .....

Table of Content

Chapter-1:- Ready to sleep?

For making a wonderful day you need to start with a wonderful morning, the secret behind a wonderful morning lies on its preparation and the preparation begins the night before. You need a proper 7-8 hours of sleep and if you have a baby he/she needs a total of 9-10 hours of sleep without any compromise.

Researches showed that effects of sleeping less than 7 hours are drastic, it's been said: **"The shorter you sleep, the shorter you live".** I truly believe this fact but its vice-versa is not true. You need to complete your daily dosage of sleep, that's all!

So what is needed to be done to make your sleep worth it and make your morning joyful,

1. Bath before you go to sleep:- A lukewarm water shower before bed is one of the most relaxing things that you should try in your life. It helps the circulation of blood all throughout your body and relaxes your mind. It relaxes you and your essential body muscle and lulls you into your bed.

2. Closing your eye and recapping your day:- It been just 2 months I'm trying this technique, through this, I have seen two

improvements within me. First, it helped to sharpen my memory and second it made me understood the worth of my day. I personally request you to try this for at least 21 days because **"work done continuously for 21 days is no more work it's a habit!"**.

3. Clean your bedsheet and pillow:- Before going to bed its a sanitary habit to clean your bedsheet and pillow because they are the companion with whom you going to spend your next 8 hours. Plus a clean environment means sound sleep.

4. Close your eyes and enter your space:- **Personally,** when I sleep, I feel like leaving this world and going to my own world. I leave everything behind, study tension, day's stress or any argument with anyone. In my world, there is always peace and calmness it's a kind of place where I can go and just relax and its always present there for me.

Chapter 2:- Sleep: -A Blessing in disguise

How many of you know the fact that **"Sleep deprivation can kill you faster than food deprivation".** Well, it's not an assumption or just simply talk in the air, it's a fact ! which should be taken seriously.

WHO along with other allied institutes of health proved that it just takes 10-15 minutes to a normal person to fall asleep. Many will argue that they keep lying in the bed for hours still they can't get good sleep, then they try to overdose themselves with sleeping pills, some tries addiction like drinking to get better sleep. Are these techniques natural, hell no!

Insomnia is a condition where a person feels frequent sleep deprivation. Although many research is been conducted in this topic but the main reason behind it is considered to be stress and anxiety. Who doesn't have stress and anxiety, but are all the insomniac ?? No. The main secret how you deal with this problem lies within your sleeping practices.

One could practice **Deep sleeping.** Well, it may seem to appear anti-advisory type because we always talk about staying alert even in our sleep which is certainly denying the fact that deep sleeping practice is good. Here lies the secret, we don't have to be in our deep sleep throughout the night deep sleep for just 1-2 hour for the adult human body is sufficient, for babes its 3-4 hours. So what is it and how can we practice it.

Deep sleep is a state of your body when you are in the deepest point in the ocean of your sleep deeply indulge in your sleep and dream. I will not say this only occurs during the darkest hours of the nights, because that's not true.

Everyone's deep sleeping programs are different. Now coming to benefits of deep sleeping

- Relaxes your tightened muscle
- Slower your heart rates
- Slows down brain waves:- Now it's a point to discuss. Through various MRI scans and modern health science tools, it was proved that brain waves are most active during the busiest hour of the day, whereas they are mostly passive during deep sleep. The more passive your brain waves are during

sleeping the more space your brain gets to repair itself.

Humans spend 1/3rd of their lives sleeping so why not just make it worth it.

It's a common belief that more money brings you more insecurity and sleep deprivation. Well, **The International Institute of sleep council** proved that **HIGH EARNERS GETS THE BEST SLEEP**, it may be due to the body's exhaustion or deep satisfaction anyway this fact proved something that money can buy sleep!

Chapter 3:- Morning Bird

Humans are only mammals that willingly delay sleep, this fact may amaze you as it did to me because many animals like sloth even sleep for 16-18 hours! That's because that is their sleep requirement. We humans don't need to sleep for more than just 8 hours.

So why can't we wake up early when our requirement is fulfilled, the answer is we have programmed our brains like that. **Dysania** is a disorder that causes us to delay our sleep in the morning and sleep for some extra hour snoozing our alarm.

Researchers have proved that condition of dysania is not innate rather its an acquired one, one which is developed through many year's malpractices.

To reverse the effect of dysania we have to follow up the reverse practice that had made up this habit within us and that's simple through various baby steps.

- Don't make drastic changes:- Deconstructing a mal-habit needs slow but steady changes, like if you wake up at 9 am every morning, suddenly you can't start waking up at 4:30 am from the very next morning. For adopting that you need to wake up the next day at 7 am, next day 6, next day 5 and so on.

- Sleep Early:- Somehow in the 24-hour schedule, you have to sleep for 8 hours, whether sleeping 2 hours in the afternoon and 6 hours in the night or sleeping 8 hours in a row, you have to complete your daily sleep dosage. For waking up at 5 am in the morning you need to straight go to bed by 9 pm or if you want to wake up by 6, 10 straight to bed!
- GO out of your bedroom as soon as you shut off your

alarm:- Everyone might be knowing this simple technique to get out of the bed in the morning like placing the alarm or your cell away from your bed so that you can leave your bed leaving a message to the body that "buddy the day has started !".Well here you can implement other simple technique that is to leave your room just go out and witness the beautiful sunrise. This technique will make your morning and you will love early waking!

- Make waking up a reward:- Every morning I wake up

early, I developed this technique, I don't know whether it is healthy or not but helped me in due course of time. As soon as I wake up I leave the bed goes to my study table open my laptop and check my Instagram feeds. It helps as a reward but I will not advise it too all as some Instagram feeds work as morning deteriorators.

- Enjoy the early dawn:- There is nothing beautiful than an early sunrise in that hour of the morning so why not witness it. Just grab your cup of coffee and go to the balcony and be a part of this beautiful nature's creation.

One way or other great leaders are early risers, just because they work when everybody else is sleeping so that they will be successful when everybody is not. So, by developing this habit of early rising you can get one step more close to that **League of leaders.**

And as always **Early bird gets the worm.**

Chapter 4:- The Rituals

Okay, we all were waiting for this, now it's here important to learn that the things we are going to discuss going to make your day.

You woke up, laziest part of your day heart wants to return back to the bed but head keeps reminding you that you need to face this day because this day is important for you and you know what **the day is actually important for you** so you just can't start it being lazy and unplanned. You need to man up get your things done and go ahead face your day **the bed will remain there waiting for you to come back that night and have a**

satisfactory sleep as you won the day!

- Morning Meditation:- The moment you wake up just leave the bed, the work of your bed is done there now its just you and your day. Get out of the room brush your teeth first get a glass of normal water and then sit somewhere quiet, I like to go to the balcony as it is the quietest place in my home. Just sit and start taking a deep breath you can take the aid of any meditation app if you like, they are great these days. Just sit and meditate for 5 minutes. Ladies and

Gentlemen, I just can't describe to you how much beautiful effect meditation leaves in your life. Researches have shown meditation actually increases the grey matter inside your brain which stores and analyses information and also involved in excellence. Give your body a sense of calmness and breathe.

- Journaling your day:- Here comes the planning part. Spartans always believed this philosophy **sharpest spear has the finest mould**. You need to produce a nice blueprint of your day following which you can win your day. So take a diary or a piece of paper and **write** everything you want to do today, **prioritize** the list then **assign** time for every work. Following the above steps, you can complete your day and always remember noting down stuff will not help you achieve your goals, it's your action towards that goal which will help you achieve it.

- Make yourself hydrated:- It's the important part of the morning that everyone ignores. **The human body is 70% water and the body**

loses 30% of its water while sleeping so to fulfill that water demand you need to hydrate yourself. I'm actually a kind of person who forgets drinking water so I developed this technique to drink lemon water while journaling, water hydrates me and the lemon juice adds electrolytes to my body.

- Exercise:- Get out of your comfort zone and do something to circulate your blood as said by great philosophers **Moving is life, stagnant is death.** Run, swim, workout weights do anything but ensure you are sweating and having a good blood circulation around your body.

- Have your breakfast:- First meal of the day is called breakfast because by having it you are breaking your 8-10 hours fast that you had unknowingly since the last night's dinner till now. So it's very important to have the first meal of the day so that it will fuel your body and get you working.

Now that you have completed your rituals, you are ready to face the day but never forget rituals are something that is meant to be done every day, so keep your pace for it every day and achieve anything you want day by day!

Chapter 5:- Man of Practice

During childhood my father made me join Karate classes, I was a regular comer there but for some reason, I hated that early morning classes then school, studies, homework lots of burden which later I realize wasn't boring just a part of the struggle.

There was a boy who came there one day, I don't remember properly but he was somewhat 7 years older than me and got a huge physique. Everyone assumed he was the perfect candidate for the December tournament. Despite his good physique which he got in inheritance he was not regular in the classes but the day he used to come sensei used to train him vigorously he also used to win every practice match just for the sake of his huge mass.

December tournament came I was also participating but no one has good expectations for me, I too stood for that guy because he was representing our institute. The fight started what we used to call Kumite, I was under 40 kg weight category and that guy was under 90 kg more than double of me. I still remember he fell like a big tree in the arena against a guy who was smaller than him. I still remember that day, that guy never came classes after that tournament. Next, when I came under 90 kg weight category I had to attain that tournament too once again I asked sensei to help me improve myself. He simply told me Raj, Idea is the captain, practice is the soldier if your captain is strong but your soldiers are weak your army will get defeated. This line made me remember that boy. I learned you can get many things from inheritance but practice and hard work are certainly not among them. Although my performance was not up to the mark, got bronze but the lesson I got was equivalent to gold.

While I was implementing these morning rituals into my life before writing this book I remembered that same session from my sensei. Today when I used to wake up at 5 am and I go for jogging I realize new dawn has something beautiful, something which brings us close to nature, something which there urban late sleeping people would never experience.

I jog through woods, through farmyards, crop fields, water canal and it feels like more distance I cover the more closer I'm getting to myself. This would have been never possible if I wouldn't consistently practice my rituals.

"Many roads lead to the path, but basically there are only two: reason and practice"

- **Bodhidharma**

Chapter 6:- End Product

At the beginning of the chapter, I wrote all the techniques and methodologies that are going to be a part of your morning from now onwards are all the techniques and ways that I have performed of my own but I never told you from where I learned all these what motivated me to perform all this.

So, from childhood itself, I was curious about all the life-changing techniques, how to master yourself, how to plan your day and all I learned many techniques. From learning I mean just getting to know stuffs but never practically applying them in my life. It was just a year ago I found myself getting lazy and drowsy. Although I used to sleep for more than nine hours but my days weren't much productive. As I told you during the beginning of the chapter I am a student and as a student with an ambition to perform well you cannot afford to be lazy during the lectures.

I was a great fan of authors who used to write about life mastery and eventually that led me to the idea that, if there is no shame in changing then there should be no shame in sharing your change with other people. Now I am here happy with my morning rituals, living a productive day and making the best ever memories that I can make in my life.

As I told earlier, ***"Moving is life and stagnant is death".*** It's one hundred percent true, remember last time you felt like you are stuck in your life that's just because you haven't adopted any change in recent. So, go ahead take a single step to change your 8 am morning routine and make yourself a 5 am person I'm sure you will start having awesome days and a collection of awesome days adds up to make an awesome life.

Chapter-7:- Conclusion

I hope my ways would be helpful for you. Before closing this book I want to share ways with my readers to ensure that this book will be of utmost use to all.

1. *Take notes from this book and jot it down in your personal journal.*
2. *Make a report of your daily progress by writing it down.*
3. *Be grateful to yourself and encourage yourself to take your life to the next level.*
4. *Reward yourself blissfully once you will complete your*

daily tasks, this will make your tasks joyful.

5. *Have trust on you and your practices.*

It's important to know that it's not possible to convince anyone before you have convinced yourself. Convince yourself that this idea will work and it will definitely help you living a better life.

Thank you, live the life you want to live!

www.ingramcontent.com/pod-product-compliance
Lightning Source LLC
Chambersburg PA
CBHW060344290526
45791CB00004B/1531